Index

Introduction

My name is Christine and I have Multiple Sclerosis. Thank you for buying this book. You will have bought it for one of many reasons; either you have Multiple Sclerosis (MS), you know someone who has or maybe you just want to know more about this very debilitating disability. Whatever your reason I hope that you will find this e-book both interesting and informative; also a little light hearted, but most of all I hope that it will convince you that **we** *can* **cope with MS no matter what it throws at us.**

What is MS?

So what is MS? Quite simply a central nervous systems disorder that attacks the brain stem and spinal column. It affects the body by gradually destroying the myelin that coats the nerve endings. Multiple Sclerosis means 'many scars' and that is exactly what happens to the myelin, the nerve endings are broken down and left with many scars. This can reduce or even stop the signals from the brain connecting to whichever part of the body you are currently trying to use. Liken this to a car with dirty spark plugs, you will get plenty of sparks but no actual ignition, it's the same with your body. Your body functions are interfered with because of a diminished or unresponsive connection between the brain and the nerve endings. Anything can be affected, sight, hearing, legs, arms and even balance. The main thing to remember is that MS

is

1. NOT a mental illness

2. NOT contagious and

3. NOT preventable or curable although there is

a lot of research going on worldwide.

What Causes MS?

There are many thoughts on this one but scientists have come up with 3 main theories.

1. Virus attack

Viruses act in different ways. Some act quickly, the common cold, whereas others take some time to show any symptoms, maybe months or years. Theory 1 says that a slow-acting virus or a delayed reaction to one of the more common ones could cause MS.

2. Immune Reaction

Our bodies are made to fight attacks from viruses and bacteria, this usually works very well. Our autoimmune system kicks in when invaded and fights the nasties but theory 2 says that in MS sufferers this may have gone wrong. Our auto-immune system can sometimes attack it's own body cells by mistake and this is called an 'auto-immune reaction'. Theory 2 says that this how MS could be triggered.

3. Combination

When viruses invade the body, they take over body cells. Theory 3 states that it is when our defense system could become confused and start to attack both virus and cell at the same time. Whilst talking to a friend at my local MS Therapy Center she said that she was told that MS could be triggered by a particularly stressful episode in your life. I don't know if this is true but it is certainly something else to consider.

Who Gets MS?

MS usually shows itself in men and women between the ages of 20 and 40. It very seldom strikes people under 15 or over 50. It is a known fact that more women than men suffer MS although it is not known why. Female MS sufferers can still have children as it is thought that pregnancy does not affect MS. Those less likely to contract MS are Polynesians, Native Americans and black South Africans. These are not the only ones but they do seem to be more resistant to MS than some other cultures. MS is also less prevalent in Tropical and sub-tropical areas.

Types of MS

When you mention MS to people, they generally think that there is only one type. To them MS is MS and that's the end of the story. Surprisingly there are three different types of MS and not all of them mean that you will be severely disabled. I will now explain how the various types will affect the sufferer.

1. Benign

Those who have this kind of MS are the most difficult do diagnose. This is because they may show no signs of having anything wrong with them for a long time, maybe 1- to 15 years. Benign MS is the kindest form of this disability, as it will produce no long-term effects. Those who have this type of MS will have a few mild attacks but will generally be very healthy individuals.

2. Relapsing/Remitting

This is the most common form that MS takes. Those with this type will be reasonably well for some time and then will suffer some form of relapse. The symptoms that are displayed by the individual will vary and may last days, weeks, months or even years. Once they have gone the sufferers, display few if any symptoms and will pretty much return to the way that they were before the relapse.

3. Progressive

Progressive MS falls into one of three categories; these are Primary, Secondary and Chronic. I will now cover each of these in more detail.

Primary Progressive MS

Displays itself as a gradual deterioration from the onset of MS, without any sudden relapses.

Approximately 10% of sufferers are Primary Progressive.

Secondary Progressive

This type of Chronic Progressive MS is usually the next stage for people who have had Relapsing/Remitting MS. They will find that their symptoms worsen gradually over time without them having had any relapses. It is possible to still have some relapses whilst experiencing this stage.

Chronic Progressive

This is the most brutal form of MS and means that the symptoms get worse and worse until the sufferer usually needs to use a wheelchair. This transition could take months or years; it is hard to say which as each person reacts to Chronic Progressive MS in a different way.

What are the Symptoms?

Now that we understand more about MS, we need to look at the symptoms. These can be varied and very disturbing to those that have them. They differ from person to person and can change each time that an individual suffers a relapse. Below is a list of some of the symptoms that someone with MS might experience.

1. Double vision, blurred vision, difficulty with focusing or uncontrolled eye movement.

2. Numbness or changed sensation to touch, heat or pain

3. Tingling feelings in the arms, legs, hands or feet

4. Complete or partial paralysis of any part of the body

5. Shaking of the hands

6. Loss of bladder or bowel control

7. Dizziness

8. Loss of balance and/or staggering

9. Speech problems, the sufferer may stutter or slur

10. Weakness or unusual tiredness

11. Difficulty in walking, the legs may feel stiff, painful or just clumsy

12. Loss of co-ordination

13. Short term memory loss

14. Difficulty in concentrating

15. Mood swings

Sufferers can get any of these symptoms, sometimes more than one at a time. In the early stages of MS, they may be hardly noticeable and not worth a visit to the doctor but, later on they could become so severe that it would be advisable to seek medical help.

There are many ways of alleviating the symptoms of MS and I will cover these later in the book.

Diagnosing MS

MS is not an easy thing to diagnose; the symptoms are so varied that they could be attributed to other diseases of the central nervous system. The symptoms of MS also come and go so you may be suffering no symptoms on the day of your examination. There is currently no laboratory test that can pinpoint MS and the most common way of trying to diagnose it is by the Magnetic Resonance Imaging (MRI) Scanner. This involves the individual concerned being put into a machine that will take photographs of the spinal column and brain stem. This is done using a high frequency electromagnetic impulse to try to spot the white lesions caused by MS. The machine is very noisy and sometimes, especially if you have a tendency to become dizzy, the doctor will be able to perform this procedure under anesthetic.

For those who are not happy lying in a long tube for about an hour the MRI scan is available at some hospitals as an upright sit in tube, still noisy but a lot more comfortable.

Another way of trying to diagnose MS is by lumbar puncture. This involves removing some of the fluid from the spinal column by inserting a needle into the gap between two of the discs at the base of the spine. Personally speaking I don't rate this idea much. When it was offered to me I flatly refused, as you need to remain flat on your back for 24 hours after the procedure is completed. If you don't you are likely to suffer severe headaches.

The best advice that I can offer is to ask many questions about the different forms of diagnosis and then decide which one you would be happiest with.

Treating MS

Because there is no current cure for MS, we have to learn how to cope with the symptoms. Fortunately many treatments are available to help alleviate the pain and discomfort caused by this disability, and keep us active. We are very lucky in the UK because we have therapy centers dotted around the country; each one is manned by professional people that are there to help. The catchphrase to remember is **'Use it or lose it'**; this brings home the importance of staying as mobile as possible. Wherever you go you will be told the importance of diet and exercise.

There are obviously some foods more beneficial than others and your dietician will advise you what you should eat to maintain a good standard of health.

Most therapy centers have a physiotherapist on site to deal with any problems associated with the muscles. They will help you perform simple stretching exercises and other movements to help with your mobility and balance. If you are lucky, your therapy center will have Hyperbolic Oxygen (HBO) tanks. These are very good for helping to combat dizziness, fatigue and numbness. I have tried this particular therapy on more than one occasion, having spent an hour in the HBO tank I emerged to feel that I could take on the world. If you get the chance this would be a good one to try. In some therapy centers, you may be offered the chance to try exercising in the water. I recommend this as the water bears your weight making any movements much easier, and much more comfortable. As far as exercise goes lots of people have said that Yoga is extremely good for those with MS. This one works because it is a gentler form of exercise with slower movements. Because you do everything at a much more sedate pace, your muscles are getting a good workout without the stresses and strains of conventional exercise. The physiotherapist can also give advice on any walking aids etc. that might be needed.

You will also find that when you are first diagnosed you will be offered the chance to talk to a councilor. This is a good idea because many different thoughts and feelings will be going through your head right now. This is normal as, if you are like me, your initial diagnosis would be a bit of a blow. You will probably have known that something was wrong but you will not have known what. The councilor will talk to you about the way you are feeling but will never tell you what to do or how to do it. He/she is simply there to let you get things off your chest; this is an invaluable service and should be used if ever things are getting too much for you.

So, apart from the Dietician, Physiotherapist and Councillor, what else is on offer? Well at my Therapy Centre they also have an MS Nurse, Speech Therapy, a Continence Nurse, Reflexology sessions, Aromatherapy massage, Shiatsu massage, Pilates exercise in or out of the pool and a toning table. Some of these incur a small charge but most are free.

That just about covers the Therapy Centre but what can the doctor do for you?

Your doctor can help in many ways. For those who suffer muscle weakness and spasms there are several different drugs available. The most talked about one of these is **Beta Interferon**. Interferons are proteins that are produced by the body in response to a foreign substance, a virus for example. Beta Interferon seems to calm the overactive immune system and has been shown to slow the progression of MS. Because this drug is so expensive it is only given to more severe cases, and also only after the Consultant's go-ahead. It can be given by injection or in tablet form but, be warned, you are not advised to drink anything like coffee as you can become permanently high as a side effect.

Another drug that can be prescribed is **Copaxone**. This one has similar effects to Beta Interferon and has to be given by injection. Sometimes you will not need such drugs and a course of **Vitamin B12**, given as an injection by your practice nurse, can be very beneficial. I have undergone a course of B12 injections and have found that they help fight fatigue. On a lighter note, did you know that B12 would also keep the bugs away in the summer? Apparently, they don't like the smell coming from your pores and will absolutely refuse to munch on you.

Because the course of MS is so unpredictable it is vital to have regular evaluations on your condition. If you go to a Therapy Center, you will probably find that they will ask you to attend a yearly assessment. You should also make a point of seeing you GP if you think that anything is wrong. He/she will be able to tell you whether it's MS or something completely different.

Living with MS

The first time that I can remember having any MS symptoms was probably about 15 years ago. It started with a loud ringing in my ears and then my head would start to spin. For a long time I was fed antibiotics because the doctor kept telling me that I had an ear infection, but then they finally realized that I seemed to be having far too many. All the help then seemed to stop until I moved to Bedford UK. Just after I moved I had another dizzy spell, only this time I collapsed in the street. It upset me that so many people just walked past and didn't even ask if I was all right, they seemed to assume that I was the worse for alcohol. I was lucky enough to be approached by an old woman who knocked on the nearest door and insisted that the owner took me home in her car. At this point, I was still feeling very ill and my GP had no idea what was wrong with me. I was sent for the usual battery of tests, blood, sugar, blood gases and many others but still nothing could be found. Then I fell pregnant with my youngest daughter and that's when the fun really started. I was working in a fast food restaurant at the time and, not only did I have to put up with the usual morning sickness, I also became more and more dizzy and had terrible hot flushes. I put this down to being pregnant as many women do have these problems. My daughter was eventually born by caesarean section and I hoped that this would mark an end to my troubles, not so. A couple of days after I came home my legs started to feel very heavy and I could not move them properly. My GP insisted that I went back into hospital for further tests, which I did. My consultant was a neurologist and seemed to delight in sticking pins into me and asking if I could feel anything. I was x-rayed to see if there was anything that they could identify and I was not allowed to get out of bed without the nurses help. Eventually the Consultant told me that he *thought* I had MS, which was only after he had considered another possibility called Meniers Disease.

After his diagnosis I went into, I suppose what can only be described as, a state of shock. All the usual questions went through my head, what is it? Why me? What have I done to get this disease? However, nothing really helped and it was my GP who really answered most of the questions for me. He also referred me to the MS Therapy Center in Bedford and I was so happy that he did. It is manned by friendly, welcoming people and is a place where you do not feel alone. I mentioned earlier some of the treatments that they have to offer and, I think, I have used most of them at some point. As MS sufferers go, I have not been too bad yes, I have had to use a stick to help me walk and yes I have had to have Steroid based injections every day for a week, but now I manage the difficulties of MS quite well. I have been retired from work on the grounds of ill health but I haven't let that stop me. I plan to study from home and write more books about the thing that I know best. Typing is difficult right now because I only have feeling in my right hand and cannot feel the keys under my fingers, but that won't stop me. Some of my friends at the Therapy Center are better than me and some are worse but, we all have one thing in common, **Positive thinking**. Without positive thinking, we all believe that we would sink into the quagmire of despair never to return. Here are some more ideas for making MS treat you more kindly;

1. Heat

Some of us are more susceptible to heat and this means that we don't have our bath or shower too hot, our heating is never on full blast and we do not tend to sit in the sun for too long. I remember a little while a go being told that it would be beneficial to try out a cold suit in the summer. These were based on suits worn by NASA spacemen to regulate body heat. Although they, apparently, worked very well the price was enough to put most people off of owning one.

Overall dealing with heat is just common sense. Take adequate precautions in the sun and check the temperature of your bath/shower before you get in. I know that a shower that is too hot for me will increase the numbness in my arms and legs so I usually ask someone to check the temperature for me. My central heating is switched off as soon as any cold snaps are gone. In this way I find that I am not as tired as usual, my symptoms are kept to a minimum and I am much happier.

2. Diet

Diet also has a very important part to play in our well-being. If we cut down on certain foods like hard cheeses, eggs and white bread we will gradually notice a difference in the way we feel. Most people use vegetable oil now for frying and this is a much healthier way of doing it. However, when it comes to MS foods like bacon, chops and even chips should be cooked in the oven, this reduces the amount of fat intake and encourages the body to be much healthier.

Some MS sufferers, myself included, endorse the benefits of Evening Primrose Oil. This is taken in capsule form and is available from your GP if requested. Vitamin B12 injections or pills are also useful for combating fatigue; these are available from your GP, practice nurse or your local pharmacy.

3. Relaxation

The best and nicest thing for you to practice is some form of relaxation. This can be anything from Yoga to just sitting down with your eyes closed listening to your favorite music. Relaxation will reduce your stress level, we all know that MS is no friend to stress, and give you a great sense of calm. There are audio tapes and CD's available with some very beautiful relaxation music on them. These range from Gregorian chant to sounds of the jungle and whale or dolphin song. Put one on, close your eyes and let your imagination take you on a wonderful journey of peace and tranquility.

4. Communication

This can be a big obstacle for some MS people at times. They seem to think that by saying how they feel they will be boring their family and friends. Not so, they care about you and if you are feeling under the weather, they may be able to help you in some way, maybe just vacuuming the floor or washing the dishes. Don't leave your GP out of the communication loop either, he/she is the one that you *need* to tell of any changes in your condition so that they know how best to deal with it. If you are working, let your employer know what's happening. Most workplaces can be very sympathetic towards disability now and they might be able to adjust your work pattern for you. You may want to decrease the hours that you work or even start later or finish earlier, a good employer will try their best to help you with this.

Closing Thought

Whatever stage your MS has reached just remember, **think positively** and **never be afraid to ask for help**. Be well and stay safe.

Acknowledgements

Dr Manford - Neurological consultant

Dr Griffith - GP

Margot and Jan - Practice Nurses

All the staff at the MS Therapy Center in Bedford

A special thank you to my family.

Thank you all, I couldn't have made it without you.

www.ingramcontent.com/pod-product-compliance
Lightning Source LLC
Chambersburg PA
CBHW070122010626
45794CB00012B/1230